HOW TO LOSE WEIGHT WITHOUT HITTING THE GYM:

The ultimate guide to losing weight without hitting the GYM.

George Hults, 2023

Table ofContents

Chapter 1

What most people don't know about health, nutrition and fitness.

Most of us do not know what healthy eating is all about: less fried food, less sugar, and more vegetables and fruits. When it comes to having proper nutrition, however, too many of us don't grasp the full intricacies of the advantages of good nutrition and how to go about getting it.

Nutrition is a crucial element of a healthy lifestyle and the significance of doing it properly cannot be stressed - let's start by diving into the advantages of having a nutritious diet. A lot of us wrongly link weight reduction with fad diets, but eating a nutritious diet is the best approach to go about maintaining a healthy weight and at the same time getting the required nutrients for optimal bodily function.

Swapping unhealthy junk food and snacks out for nutritious food is the first step to maintaining your weight within a healthy range according to your body composition, without the need to jump on the fad-diet bandwagon.

Many chronic illnesses such as type-2 diabetes and heart disease are induced by poor diet and obesity. With 1 in 9 Singaporeans suffering from diabetes, the focus on excellent eating is greater than ever. Taking a preventative approach with a whole food-based nutrition plan also minimizes the chance of acquiring other associated disorders such as renal failure.

Our immune system needs vital vitamins and minerals to operate efficiently. Eating a balanced and diverse diet guarantees your immune system performs at top capacity and defends against infections and immunodeficiency disorders. Certain kinds of food such as tomatoes and berries may promote vitality and improve cognitive function, all the while safeguarding your body against the consequences of aging.

Eating the correct meals may make you happy — minerals such as iron and omega-3 fatty acids present in a protein-rich diet can increase your mood. This helps to higher overall mental well-being and protects you against mental health disorders.

Managing portion sizes is all about ensuring that you are receiving the proper quantities of nutrients and calories from your diet. Over-eating or under-eating deprives you of nutrients and might impact your weight, so always manage your meal quantities. When purchasing food, look out for the serving sizes on the nutrition labels to determine what corresponds to a standard portion and how much it delivers in terms of nutrients.

Fresh, whole foods are the ones you will gain the greatest nutritional advantages from. Always aim for items in their purest, unadulterated form such as fresh fruits, vegetables, and meat wherever feasible. If you go with processed alternatives, consider ones that have undergone minor alterations like dehydration and flash freezing to reduce nutritional loss.

Also, keep an eye on the ingredients list to ensure that you're ingesting as few additives with your meal as possible. Consider balancing your salt consumption with other herbs and spices to provide a new layer of taste to your cuisine. For example, basil, garlic, paprika, and cayenne may transform an average chicken breast meal into a gastronomical treat.

Salt is the most frequent food ingredient used in cooking, however too much salt may contribute to high blood pressure and hypertension, especially in individuals who are already prone to those disorders. Maintaining a healthy eating plan is easy enough; analyzing if it's nutritious enough may be uncomplicated as well.

A well-structured dietary plan should enable a person to maintain a healthy physique within acceptable body fat levels (18-24% for males and 25-31% for women). This also implies that it should promote metabolic health via numerous mechanisms, such as supporting healthy hormone function, insulin sensitivity, and physical recovery.

Monitoring your cholesterol levels and blood pressure is vital since having a healthy weight doesn't reduce the likelihood of complications in these areas. While dietary cholesterol doesn't have as much impact on blood cholesterol levels as we formerly assumed, it may still be affected by your total dietary fat consumption. On the other end, high salt consumption may lead to hyper-extension, of which one of the indications occurs be raised blood pressure levels.

The state of your skin and hair are reliable indications of the quality of your diet. If you are receiving adequate nutrients, your skin should be firm, elastic, and of a deep color rather than flaky and pallid. Your hair should be silky and robust rather than dry and brittle; unexplained hair loss is generally an indication of starvation.

Getting the correct number of nutrients and calories can help you remain energetic owing to its capacity to promote peaceful sleep. If you find yourself feeling sluggish, It might be a symptom of either a definite shortage of calories and/or nutrients, forcing your body into famine mode which limits its repairing powers.

Your bowel motions indicate whether you are receiving adequate fiber from your diet, so if you find yourself being constipated, load up on extra fruits and veggies to get your digestive system flowing.

Chapter 2

Eating the right Meal.

Eating a healthy diet is not about rigid constraints, keeping excessively slim, or depriving yourself of the things you enjoy.
Rather, it's about feeling fantastic, having more energy, enhancing your health, and raising your attitude.

Healthy eating does not have to be unduly difficult. If you feel overwhelmed by all the contradicting nutrition and diet advice out there, you're not alone. It appears that for every expert who advises you a specific cuisine is beneficial for you, you'll find another claiming precisely the opposite.
The fact is that although certain single meals or minerals have been proven to have a good influence on mood, is your overall dietary pattern that is most significant.

Cooking more meals at home may help you take responsibility for what you're eating and better manage precisely what goes into your food. You'll consume fewer calories and avoid the chemical additives, added sugar, and harmful fats in packaged and takeaway meals that may leave you feeling fatigued, bloated, and irritated, and worsen symptoms of melancholy, stress, and anxiety.

What to go for \sWhole grains.
Whole-grain meals such as brown rice and bread are kinds of carbohydrates, especially unprocessed carbs. They supply you with energy, nutritious fiber, vitamins, minerals, and antioxidants, and assist with digestion.

For people who are diagnosed with coeliac or those with non-coeliac gluten sensitivity, you must include other carbohydrate alternatives to ensure that your abstinence from wheat doesn't cost you in terms of essential nutrients.

Gluten-free carbohydrate options include rice products, buckwheat (technically a pseudocereal), quinoa, and starchy vegetables (e.g. sweet potato, yam, pumpkin, maize) (e.g. sweet potato, yam, pumpkin, corn).
Fruits and veggies.

Various forms of produce are rich sources of vitamins and minerals that help regulate body functions and protect it against chronic diseases. To get the most nutrients out of your fruits and veggies, eat them whole - for example, consume entire fruits instead of having them juiced.

Protein is the key food responsible for creating and repairing muscle tissue in the body. Animal meat is the most prevalent source of protein, but there are also various plant-based sources to pick from such as nuts and legumes.

Individuals on plant-based diets should ensure they consume the proper balance of plant protein to ensure that their nutritional demands are sufficiently addressed.

Dietary fat (such as the sort you receive from fish and olive oil) is vital for optimum health as they manage cholesterol levels in your body while boosting healthy cell activity.

Monounsaturated, polyunsaturated, and saturated fat all have a part in this element of optimal health. On the other hand, the extra fat you commonly find in fried meals should be limited since they are mostly polyunsaturated fat obtained from processed vegetable oils such as soybean and rapeseed.

Due to their low threshold for oxidization, overconsumption of polyunsaturated fat may lead to inflammatory conditions and the generation of free radicals. Artificial trans fat is likewise a definite no-no.

Sugar should also be controlled — although the natural sugars available in fruits and whole grains are beneficial, the refined variety you get with cakes and snacks may alter your weight and contribute to metabolic illnesses if ingested in excess.

Eating foods rich in dietary fiber (grains, fruit, vegetables, nuts, and beans) may help you keep regular and lessen your risk for heart disease, stroke, and diabetes. It can also improve your skin and even help you to lose weight.

As well as leading to osteoporosis, not getting enough calcium in your diet can also contribute to anxiety, depression, and sleep difficulties.

Whatever your age or gender, it's crucial to incorporate calcium-rich foods in your diet, avoid those that deplete calcium, and obtain enough magnesium and vitamins D and K to help calcium do its work.

Carbohydrates are one of your body's key sources of energy. But the majority should come from complex, unprocessed carbohydrates (vegetables, whole grains, fruit) rather than sweets and refined carbs.

Chapter 3

Proper Meal Timing.

We need a certain amount of energy each day, and at different times throughout the day, to thrive. This energy comes from the carbs, fats, and proteins we consume.

Regular meals and snacks allow for more opportunities in the day to give our body the energy and nutrients it needs to function optimally, allowing us to engage in all the things we need to do in the day.

Ever feel drained by 3 pm and ready to take a nap? This might be your body's natural response to having gone multiple hours (since lunch) without a re-up of energy.

When we do not eat enough times in the day, for example, if we only eat one or two meals per day, it can be quite difficult to meet our energy and nutritional needs (e.g. protein, calcium, iron, fiber).

If you have pretty reliable hunger cues, you might notice that your body tries to make up for it when you don't eat enough during the day. For example, skipping breakfast may result in increased cravings in the afternoon and/or evening to make up for the lack of energy consumed earlier in the day.

Skipping an afternoon snack might result in being overly hungry, eating more quickly, and possibly eating past your comfortable fullness level at dinner time.

Regular meal timing also helps to promote regular digestion. Going extended periods without eating can increase our likelihood of eating more quickly or eating more than we may need at our next meal, which can negatively impact digestion.

On the other hand, grazing continuously throughout the day prevents your body's migrating motor complex (MMC) from firing. The MMC is an electromechanical wave of muscle contractions through your gut that acts to sweep through leftover undigested food.

When we eat continuously, this housekeeper is unable to do its job and the build-up of residue can lead to increased bloating for some people.
The light/dark cycles of the day and our feeding/fasting times also affect our natural circadian rhythms.

Consistent meal timing has been shown to promote regular circadian rhythms. Studies have shown that people with irregular eating patterns may have more difficulties processing insulin and may experience increased inflammation.

There are so many articles out there promoting prolonged fasting to clear up cellular debris, promote insulin sensitivity and improve other metabolic markers.

However, it's important to note that we all naturally fast each night, from whenever we finish our evening snack to when we have breakfast in the morning, and this is when your body will shift gears from its fed to fasted state and will naturally experience those metabolic benefits that are talked about.

I recommend having something to eat within 2 hours of waking up in the morning. This will break your fast from overnight and provide your body fuel to start the day.

When we wake up and ask our bodies to engage in work meetings, getting kids ready, a morning workout, and more, without providing it any fuel to do so, it has to try to get by in its fasted state.

This will result in either feeling more tired/less energized and/or it will seek ways to get that energy eventually, for example through increased cravings or an increased pleasure reward from food later in the day.

You may find that you were never hungry in the morning, which makes sense because your body has turned down your hunger cues overnight in its powered-down state.

Regardless, I encourage you to try to have something small as it is still important to try to give your body some form of nourishment. It is important to note that caffeine also suppresses appetite, so if you find that you're fine with just a coffee in the morning, that alone may be killing your drive to eat actual food and get actual energy.

After the first meal of the day, depending on what was had and how balanced it was, most people find that they need to eat again every 3-4 hours or so. Including a protein-rich food, high-fiber starches, veg/fruits, and fats in your meals will likely result in feeling full and satisfied for longer.

Whereas a smaller, less-balanced meal might only keep you satisfied for an hour or so. Regardless of how long it's been since you've last eaten if you're hungry, you need to eat.

Sample Meal Schedule

6 am: Wake up

7-8 am: Breakfast

10-10:30 am: Morning Snack

12-1 pm: Lunch

3-4 pm: Afternoon Snack

7-8 pm: Dinner

10 pm: Bedtime

Chapter 4

The 6 scientific laws of healthy weight loss.

Some of the weight reduction articles out there these days are becoming a touch nutty. New scientific studies that provide insight on how metabolism works are excellent and essential in their own right, but when discoveries become converted into miraculous new advice for losing weight, something is awry.

Some recent papers in major publications, which have endeavored to debunk the misconceptions of weight reduction and the particular diets themselves, imply that the medical establishment is likewise becoming weary of the hoopla and the erroneous assumptions that dominate the public conversation.

When it comes down to it, the things we know to be true regarding weight reduction are quite straightforward and surely few. They are also incredibly effective when carried out.

So, from the academics who have researched this stuff for decades, here's pretty much all we know about weight reduction today, distilled down to six principles regarding how the body grows, sheds and maintains its weight.

1. Dieting trumps exercising.
We hear a lot that a little activity is a key to weight reduction - that climbing the stairs instead of the elevator will make a difference, for instance.

Decreasing food consumption is far more effective than increasing physical exercise to accomplish weight reduction. If you want to establish a 300 kcal energy deficit you may run in the park for 3 miles or not eat 2 ounces of potato chips.

Some research have proven up this duality, pitting exercise against food and found that individuals prefer to lose more weight by dieting than by exercise alone.

Of course, both combined would be much better. The trouble is that when you depend on exercise alone, it generally backfires, for a handful of reasons.

This is largely due of exercise's impact on the hunger and appetite hormones, which make you feel notably hungrier after exercise.

For every action there's a response; that's a rule of physics, not of biology, but it appears that it also operates in biological systems. This is why we frequently exaggerate very significantly an impact of a certain therapy.

The second difficulty with exercise without dieting is that it's just taxing, and again, the body will compensate. If the activity makes you fatigued enough that you become more inactive the remainder of the day, you could not suffer any net negative energy.

Some of the calories we burn come from our fundamental motions throughout the day - so if you're tired out after exercise, and more inclined to rest on the sofa afterward, you've lost the energy deficit you acquired from your jog.

2. Exercise may help restore a damaged metabolism, particularly during maintenance.
Within a few of days of non-activity, the metabolism becomes rigid. You start moving again, and it does start to alter.

Your metabolism may not ever get back to normal(more on this below), but the data shows that it may certainly start up again, in large part via exercising your body every day.

This is a significant part of why exercise is necessary in the maintenance phase, which is generally acknowledged to be more difficult than the weight reduction phase.

Exercise is very, very crucial for keeping lost weight, and persons who are not physically active are more prone to acquire weight.

We believe it's partially because, with the additional calories burnt from physical activity, you have a little more flexibility in food intake, so you're not so much depending on ridged adjustments in eating habits; it makes it more acceptable.

3. You're going to have to work harder than other people — maybe forever.
Though exercise may assist fix a metabolism that's been out of sync for a long time, the grim fact is that it may not ever get back to what it was before you acquired weight.

So if you've been overweight or obese and you lose weight, sustaining that loss means you're probably going to have to work more than other individuals, maybe for good.

The terrible part is that after you've been fat or not moving for some time, it requires a bit more activity to sustain.

Building muscle may help your body burn a few more calories throughout the day, but it's also possible that you'll have to work more aerobically in the long term.

4. There is no magical mix of meals.
We frequently imagine that if we can simply uncover the correct mix of meals, we suddenly lose weight or retain what we've lost.

There are low-fat diets, low-carb diets, low glycemic diets, paleo diets, and a lot of permutations of all of these.

5. A calorie IS a calorie.
And for energy balance, it's the quantity of calories that counts. It's absolutely true - at least in principle and occasionally in reality – that all calories are created equal.

You may gain weight by eating too much nutritious food as well as bad. From the aspect of health, it is best to consume your vegetable. It is simply a lot simpler to consume calories from junk food than from nutritious meals.

The food business has carved out a whole new branch of food science to explore the bliss point, in which meals are produced to raise the quantity it takes to feel content and full.

6. it is all about the brain.
When it comes down to it, it is not the body or the metabolism that is causing overweight or obesity — it's the brain.

We all know instinctively that bad choices are what make you gain weight and excellent ones are what help you lose it.

The trouble is that over time, the bad choices lead to profound changes in how the brain manages – and, remarkably, reacts to – the hunger and satiation processes.

Years of any form of behavior habit build down brain footprints, and overeating is no exception.
The good news is that there's emerging evidence that the brain can, in large part, correct itself if new behavior patterns form (i.e., calorie restriction, healthy food choices, and exercise) (i.e., calorie restriction, healthy food choices, and exercise).

While there may be some degree of harm to the brain, especially in how hunger and satiety hormones act, it may repair itself to a considerable degree over time.

The point is that the process does take time, and like any other habit change, is eventually a practice.

So reducing it down even further: lower calories, eat healthier, exercise, and most of all, remember that is a discipline that needs to be done over time - months or years.

The reality that you'll have to work more at maintenance than your never-overweight best buddy is disheartening, but it is worth coming to grips with.

And, most essential to remember, your brain (the organ underlying all this, after all) is malleable, and it will react to the adjustments you make — better than you imagine. And so will your body.

Chapter 5

The code of a good training partner/How to prevent workout injuries.

A training partner may be a wonderful tool in so many ways. He can spot you on exercises, such as the squat and bench press, as well as aid with forced reps, enabling you to carry large weights you couldn't quite do on your own. He can also bring encouragement and fellowship. It's a terrific feeling: to share objectives and work as a team to exceed barriers of strength and endurance.

Find someone as dedicated as you are, someone who shares similar aims to yours. If your partner jokes about when you're psyching up for a huge set, you're certain to feel upset! He should share your enthusiasm for training.

Your companion should be selfless to the core. If you need a spotter and your partner is too preoccupied checking himself out in a mirror, then I'd advocate finding a new collaboration. You want to be with someone who focuses on you when you're doing your sets, not himself.
Make sure your spouse is someone you enjoy and get along with.

You are going to be spending a large lot of time with this individual under some pretty difficult conditions. If there's too much tension between the two of you, you're not going to enjoy your time spent at the gym. And if you're not enjoying your gym time, well, you're missing the purpose. Keeping these factors in mind, you may now examine possible mates carefully.

As much as training companions might be a fantastic asset, they can also inhibit your growth. What if your spouse feels like crap? That bad energy might flow over into your exercise. Be aware of this scenario: "I'm not up for training today.

Let's go have a burger." Or "Man, I got into a major argument with my girlfriend last night. I'm not sure whether we should split up or remain together." So he's preparing to shoot himself, and you're somehow meant to enjoy your set of bench presses. No way! Never let a relationship bring you down. The aim is to be inspired, not distracted, by your companion.

Remember, good energy produces positive energy; it brings out the best in others. If you do your research and locate the proper training partner, then the sky's the limit in your training and eventually in your success as a bodybuilder.

If you're following a workout from a magazine, video, app, or general web programming, know that such routines are meant for a broad audience. You may need to follow the modification model or perhaps regress the workouts further depending on your fitness level or take more breaks than specified or a longer rest time.

Perform not doing the same program or workouts every single day. Mix up your week with routines such as upper body blast, lower body hit, and aerobic exercises. Avoid completing programs that target the same muscles and identical exercises on back-to-back days. By mixing things up you are continuously working various muscles and not over-employing the same movement patterns that may lead to overuse issues.

Strength exercises should not be unpleasant. That old saying "no pain, no gain" does not apply here. Moving in ways that give you pain is not healthy and may lead to many musculoskeletal issues either now or on the road. If you encounter discomfort during a certain workout, stop performing it and seek expert help.

It is easy to become overwhelmed when you're beginning an exercise regimen on your own. You may have concerns about form, technique, what equipment to use, how to obtain results, or simply how to stretch. If you want to work out at home but don't know where to start, an exercise physiologist is a fantastic specialist to start with.

They provide fitness tests and home workout plans that give you a thorough, whole-body fitness program with just what you need to begin began and how to advance once you have the hang of it.

Many injuries arise when we are thirsty or fatigued. Dehydration might show up as muscular spasms, cramps, dizziness, or light-headedness. And all of this may lead to harm if left uncontrolled. Always seek expert care if you acquire these symptoms or if you have prolonged discomfort after discontinuing an exercise regimen.

Taking days off is not a recommendation; it is a need for strength increases and injury avoidance. The same muscles that generate a stronger, more powerful person are also the ones that assist avoid accidents.

If they are not able to recuperate and mend from the strain of exercise, they are not growing stronger and may not be able to assist avoid injuries either. Recovery comes with sufficient water, nourishment, stretching, rest, and sleep.

Remember, you are producing good changes in your musculoskeletal system on those rest days. Even though you do not feel pain, you are training new muscles are functioning, and avoiding injuries is crucial.

Even if you're gung-ho, paying attention to your body's reaction to exercise is vital for preventing injury.

Chapter 6

How to prevent overweight permanently.

The fact is there is no "one size fits all" strategy for sustainable healthy weight reduction. What works for one person may not work for you, as our systems react differently to various diets, depending on heredity and other health considerations.

Discover the approach of weight reduction that's suitable for you will likely take time and need patience, dedication, and some experimenting with various meals and diets.

While some individuals react well to tracking calories or similar restrictive strategies, others respond well to having more latitude in organizing their weight-loss regimens.

Being free to just avoid fried meals or cut down on processed carbohydrates might set them up for success. So, don't be too disheartened if a diet that worked for someone else doesn't work for you.

And don't beat yourself up if a diet is too restricted for you to stay with. Ultimately, a diet is only good for you if it's one you can stay with over time.

Remember although there's no fast remedy to losing weight, there are lots of measures you can take to build a better connection with food, prevent emotional triggers to overeating, and attain a healthy weight.

Weight reduction is not a linear occurrence over time. When you limit calories, you may shed weight for the first few weeks, for example, and then something changes.

You consume the same amount of calories yet you lose less weight or no weight at all. That's because as you lose weight you're shedding water and lean tissue as well as fat, your metabolism slows, and your body alters in other ways.
So, to continue lowering weight each week, you need to continue reducing calories.

A calorie isn't necessarily a calorie. Eating 100 calories of high fructose corn syrup, for example, might have a different impact on your body than eating 100 calories of broccoli.

The answer for sustained weight reduction is to discard the items that are rich with calories but don't make you feel full (like sweets) and replace them with foods that fill you up without being heavy with calories (like veggies) (like vegetables).

Many of us don't always eat just to satisfy hunger. We frequently resort to eating for consolation or to ease stress—which may swiftly derail any weight reduction effort.

An alternate way of approaching weight reduction sees the issue as not one of taking too many calories, but rather the way the body stores fat after ingesting carbohydrates—in particular the impact of the hormone insulin.

When you consume a meal, carbohydrates from the food enter your circulation as glucose. To keep your blood sugar levels in control, your body always burns off this glucose before it burns off fat after a meal.

If you consume a carbohydrate-rich meal (plenty of pasta, rice, bread, or French fries, for example), your body produces insulin to deal handle the rush of all this glucose into your blood.

As well as managing blood sugar levels, insulin does two things: It blocks your fat cells from releasing fat for the body to burn as fuel (since it aims to burn off the glucose) and it generates additional fat cells for storing anything that your body can't burn off.

The upshot is that you gain weight and your body now needs more fuel to burn, so you eat more. Since insulin primarily burns carbohydrates, you need carbs and thus start a vicious cycle of ingesting carbs and gaining weight. To reduce weight, the logic goes, you need to disrupt this loop by limiting carbohydrates.

Most low-carb diets suggest replacing carbohydrates with protein and fat, which might have some detrimental long-term impacts on your health.

If you do follow a low-carb diet, you may lower your risks and limit your consumption of saturated and trans fats by selecting lean meats, fish, and vegetarian sources of protein, low-fat dairy products, and eating lots of leafy green and non-starchy vegetables.

if you don't want to gain fat, do not consume fat. Walk down any grocery store aisle and you'll be assaulted with reduced-fat snacks, dairy, and packed meals. But as our low-fat alternatives have expanded, so have obesity rates. So, why haven't low-fat diets worked for more of us?

Unsaturated fats found in avocados, nuts, seeds, soy milk, tofu, and fatty fish may help fill you full, while adding a little excellent olive oil to a plate of veggies, for example, can make it easier to consume nutritious food and enhance the overall quality of your diet.

We frequently make incorrect trade-offs. Many of us make the mistake of substituting fat for the empty calories of sugar and processed carbs. Instead of eating whole-fat yoghurt, for example, we consume low- or no-fat variants that are laden with sugar to make up for the loss of flavor.

Eating excellent fats and good carbohydrates coupled with huge quantities of fresh fruits and vegetables, nuts, seafood, and olive oil—and just small portions of meat and cheese.

All too frequently, we resort to food when we're upset or concerned, which may derail any diet and pack on the pounds. Recognizing your emotional eating triggers may make all the difference in your weight-loss attempts.

Stop eating before you are full. It takes time for the signal to reach your brain that you've had enough. Don't feel pressured to constantly clear your plate. Permanent weight reduction entails making healthy adjustments to your lifestyle and dietary choices. To keep motivated:

Set objectives to keep you motivated. Short-term objectives, like wanting to fit into a bikini for the summer, typically don't work as well as wanting to feel more confident or get healthier for your children's sake. When temptation comes, reflect on the rewards you'll get from becoming healthy.

Use tools to monitor your progress. Smartphone applications, activity monitors, or just maintaining a notebook may help you keep track of the food you consume, the calories you burn, and the weight you lose. Seeing the outcomes in black and white might help you remain motivated.

Get lots of sleep. Lack of sleep increases your appetite so you desire more food than usual; at the same time, it prevents you from feeling content, making you want to keep eating. Sleep deprivation may also influence your motivation, so aim for eight hours of decent sleep a night.

Whether or not you're deliberately intending to limit carbs, most of us eat excessive levels of sugar and refined carbohydrates such as white bread, pizza dough, pasta, pastries, white flour, white rice, and sweetened morning cereals.

Replacing refined carbohydrates with their whole-grain equivalents and removing candies and pastries is just half of the issue, however. Sugar is concealed in meals as varied as canned soups and vegetables, spaghetti sauce, margarine, and many reduced-fat foods.

Since your body receives everything it needs from sugar naturally present in meals, all these extra sugar amounts to nothing but a lot of empty calories and dangerous increases in your blood glucose.

Less sugar may yield a smaller waistline
Calories gained from fructose (found in sugary drinks such as soda and processed meals like doughnuts, muffins, and candies) are more likely to contribute to fat around your abdomen. Cutting less on sugary meals may imply a thinner waistline as well as a decreased risk of diabetes.

Even if you're lowering calories, it doesn't always imply you have to consume less food. High-fiber meals such as fruit, vegetables, legumes, and whole grains are bigger in volume and take longer to digest, making them filling—and wonderful for weight loss.

It's normally safe to eat as much fresh fruit and non-starchy veggies as you want—you'll feel full before you've overdone it on the calories. Eat veggies raw or steamed, not fried or breaded, and garnish them with herbs and spices or a little olive oil for taste.

Add fruit to low-sugar cereal—blueberries, strawberries, and sliced bananas. You'll still enjoy tons of sweetness, but with fewer calories, less sugar, and more fiber.
Bulk up sandwiches by adding nutritious vegetable options like lettuce, tomatoes, sprouts, cucumbers, and avocado.

Add additional vegetables to your favorite main dishes to make your meal more substantial. Even spaghetti and stir-fries may be diet-friendly if you use fewer noodles and more veggies. Start your dinner with salad or vegetable soup to help fill you up so you eat less of your entrée.

Cook your meals at home. This enables you to manage both portion size and what goes into the dish. Restaurant and commercial meals often have a lot more sugar, bad fat, and calories than food made at home—plus the portion sizes tend to be higher.

Serve yourself in lesser quantities. Use tiny dishes, bowls, and cups to make your quantities look bigger. Don't eat out of huge dishes or straight from food packages, which makes it harder to estimate how much you've eaten.

Eating a bigger, nutritious breakfast will jump-start your metabolism, stop you from feeling hungry throughout the day, and allow you more time to burn off the calories.
Plan your meals and snacks ahead of time. You may build your little quantity snacks in plastic bags or containers. Eating on a schedule can assist you to avoid eating when you aren't hungry.

Drink more water. Thirst may easily be mistaken for hunger, so by drinking water you can prevent unnecessary calories. Limit the number of enticing meals you keep at home. If you share a kitchen with non-dieters, keep decadent items out of sight. The degree to which exercise promotes weight reduction is up to argue, but the advantages go much beyond burning calories.

Exercise may raise your metabolism and improve your outlook—and it's something you can benefit from right now. Go for a stroll, stretch, and move about and you'll have more energy and drive to tackle the remaining tasks in your weight-loss program.

Find an exercise you like. Try strolling with a buddy, dancing, hiking, cycling, playing Frisbee with a dog, enjoying a pickup game of basketball, or playing activity-based video games with your kids.

Chapter 7

Amazing weight loss result.

Switching to a healthy diet doesn't have to be an all-or-nothing approach. You don't have to be perfect, you don't have to fully remove things you love, and you don't have to alter everything all at once—that generally simply leads to straying or giving up on your new eating plan.

When cutting down on bad items in your diet, it's crucial to replace them with healthier alternatives. Replacing hazardous trans fats with good fats (such as substituting fried chicken for grilled salmon) can make a beneficial influence on your health. Replacing animal fats for refined carbs, however (such as switching your morning bacon for a doughnut), won't decrease your risk for heart disease or increase your mood.

It's crucial to be conscious of what's in your food since manufacturers frequently conceal enormous quantities of sugar or bad fats in packaged food, even those professing to be healthy.
Focus on how you feel after eating. This will help create healthy new habits and preferences.

The healthier the food you consume, the better you'll feel after a meal. The more junk food you consume, the more likely you are to feel uncomfortable, sick, or depleted of energy.
Drink lots of water.

Water helps cleanse our bodies of waste products and toxins, but many of us go through life dehydrated—causing weariness, poor energy, and headaches. It's possible to confuse thirst for hunger, so being properly hydrated can also help you make wiser meal choices.

What is moderation? In essence, it means consuming only as much food as your body requires. You should feel satiated after a meal, but not full. For many of us, moderation means eating less than we do presently.

But it doesn't mean removing the foods you enjoy. Eating bacon for breakfast once a week, for example, may be deemed moderation if you follow it with a nutritious lunch and dinner—but not if you follow it with a box of doughnuts and a sausage pizza.

When you exclude specific meals, it's normal to crave those items more, and then feel like a failure if you give in to temptation. Start by lowering portion sizes of unhealthy meals and not eating them as frequently.

As you minimize your consumption of unhealthy foods, you may find yourself desiring them less or thinking of them as simply occasional treats. Think smaller servings. Serving sizes have risen lately. When eating out, pick an appetizer instead of an entrée, share a meal with a companion, and don't order supersized anything.

At home, visual clues may aid with portion proportions. Your dish of meat, fish, or poultry should be the size of a deck of cards and half a cup of mashed potato, rice, or pasta is roughly the size of a standard light bulb.

By presenting your meals on smaller plates or in bowls, you might mislead your brain into believing it's a bigger piece. If you don't feel satiated after a meal, add additional leafy greens or cap out the meal with fruit. Take your time. It's vital to slow down and think about food as sustenance rather than simply something to guzzle down in between meetings or on the way to pick up the kids.

It takes a few minutes for your brain to signal to your body that it has eaten enough food, so eat carefully and stop eating before you feel full. Eat with people whenever possible. Eating alone, particularly in front of the TV or computer, frequently leads to mindless overeating.

Limit snack foods in the house. Be cautious with the meals you have at hand. It's tougher to eat in moderation if you have unhealthy snacks and indulgences at the ready. Instead, surround yourself with healthy alternatives and when you're ready to reward yourself with a special treat, go out and purchase it then.

Control emotional eating. We don't always eat solely to satisfy hunger. Many of us also resort to food to reduce stress or deal with negative feelings such as melancholy, loneliness, or boredom. But by learning healthy methods to handle stress and emotions, you may recover control over the food you consume and your moods.

Eat breakfast, and eat smaller meals throughout the day. A good breakfast may boost your metabolism while eating short, balanced meals keeps your energy up all day.

Try to eat supper early and fast for 14-16 hours till breakfast the following morning. Studies show that eating just when you're most active and giving your digestive system a significant pause each day may assist to control weight.

Fruit and vegetables are low in calories and nutrient-rich, which means they are filled with vitamins, minerals, antioxidants, and fiber. Focus on eating the required daily quantity of at least five servings of fruit and vegetables and it will naturally fill you full and help you cut less on harmful items.

A serving is half a cup of raw fruit or veg or a small apple or banana, for example. Most of us need to increase the amount we now consume. Eat a medley of sweet fruit—oranges, mangos, pineapple, grapes—for dessert.

Instead of consuming manufactured snack foods, nibble on veggies such as carrots, snow peas, or cherry tomatoes together with a spicy hummus dip or peanut butter. While simple salads and steamed vegetables may quickly become monotonous, there are lots of ways to add flavor to your vegetable meals.

Add color. Not only can brighter, deeper-colored veggies offer greater quantities of vitamins, minerals, and antioxidants, but they may modify the taste and make meals more aesthetically attractive. Add color with fresh or sundried tomatoes, glazed carrots or beets, roasted red cabbage wedges, yellow squash, or sweet, colorful peppers.

Naturally sweet vegetables—such as carrots, beets, sweet potatoes, yams, onions, bell peppers, and squash—add sweetness to your meals and lessen your cravings for extra sugar. Add them to soups, stews, or pasta sauces for a pleasant sweet kick. Cook green beans, broccoli, Brussels sprouts, and asparagus in innovative ways. Instead of boiling or steaming these healthful sides, try grilling, roasting, or pan-frying them with chili flakes, garlic, shallots, mushrooms, or onion. Or marinate in tart lemon or lime before cooking.

Losing weight too rapidly may take a toll on your mind and body, making you feel sluggish, fatigued, and ill. Aim to drop one to two pounds a week so you're reducing fat rather than water and muscle.